Irritable Bowel *Syndrome*

Symptoms, Causes and Natural Relief From IBS

Ron Kness

Published by:

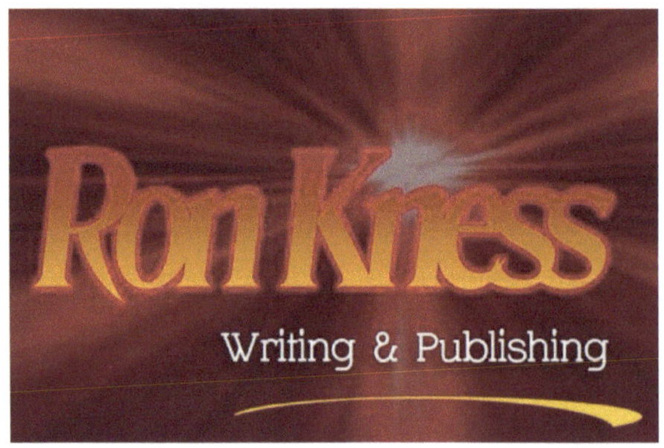

https://ronknesswriting.com

Ron Kness

Gold Canyon, AZ

United States of America

Irritable Bowel Syndrome

Disclaimer

We hope you enjoy reading this publication, however we do suggest you read our disclaimer. All the material written in this document is provided for informational purposes only and is general in nature.

Every person is a unique individual and what has worked for some or even many may not work for you. Any information perceived as advice must be considered in light of your own particular set of circumstances.

The author or person sharing this information does not assume any responsibility for the accuracy or outcome of your use of the content.

Every attempt has been made to provide well researched and up to date content at the time of writing. Now all the legalities have been taken care of, please enjoy the content.

Introduction

Irritable Bowel Syndrome or IBS is one of those horrible conditions (for sufferers) that are considered by some to be not a 'real disease'. While the symptoms vary from patient to patient, they are very real indeed for those experiencing them.

It can seem to sufferers that are diagnosed with IBS, that in the absence of being diagnosed with something more injurious to health, all that is left is an 'irritable bowel'.

The great take-away, at least, from a diagnosis of IBS, is that the symptoms experienced are not indicative of something worse, as these symptoms can certainly mimic those of other diseases.

If a diagnosis of IBS is confirmed, the next obvious step is managing, alleviating, reducing or ideally eliminating the painful and discomforting symptoms.

This eBook provides some understanding of the causes and symptoms of Irritable Bowel Syndrome. Even better, it describes natural solutions that have worked for others to provide ongoing relief.

Is It Irritable Bowel Syndrome (IBS)?

Irritable bowel syndrome is a medical condition that affects the large intestine and is known to affect around 10 to 15% of the population worldwide. This chronic gastrointestinal disorder occurs 50% more often in women than men.

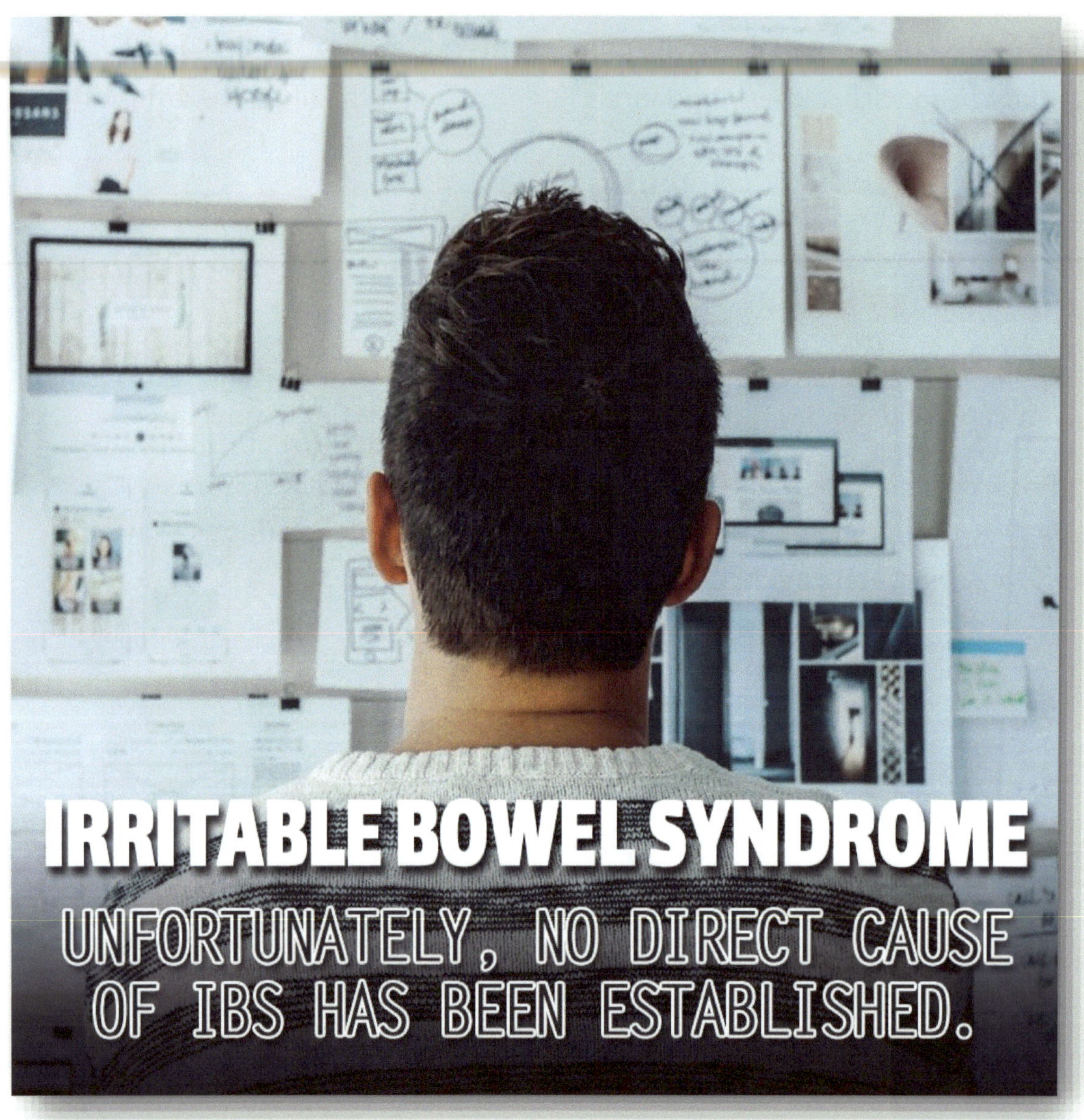

In more than half the cases of IBS the onset has occurred before 35 years of age and affects 5 % to 20% of children.

IBS is a condition belonging to a range of complaints identified as functional gastrointestinal disorders. Even though tests indicate that no abnormalities exist, the bowel still functions abnormally.

Contributing Factors

No direct cause of IBS has been established. However, researchers believe they have discovered numerous factors that may trigger the onset of symptoms. Some of these include emotional stress such as depression and anxiety, hormonal issues, some medications and digestive tract infections.

Recent studies suggest that not one but a combination of issues acting on the intestines may be responsible for IBS. Various issues relating to the intestinal wall may activate reactions that alter bowel function.

Also, bowel irritations caused by badly digested food may stimulate the nerves in the intestinal wall. This can result in intestinal sensitivity and pain.

The symptoms of IBS appear to happen because of an abnormal communication between the nervous system and the bowel.

The Connection between the Brain and the Gastrointestinal Tract (GI)

Some researchers believe that a faulty gut–brain connection may be one reason for IBS symptoms. The brain has a direct effect on the stomach ... on the whole body for that matter. And the gastrointestinal tract (GI) is sensitive to all emotions.

Feelings of anger, anxiety, sadness and even elation activate a response in the gut. Therefore, intestinal distress could be the result of feelings of anxiety, depression or other emotions. This is believed to cause abnormal muscle contractions leading to IBS symptoms

The Importance of Serotonin

There is also a belief that a lack of the neurotransmitter serotonin, may be an important trigger in the symptoms of IBS. Research has found a deficiency of serotonin in the body alters the function of the nerve cells in the bowel. This changes sensation and bowel function.

Serotonin affects our happiness, feelings and emotions, and is an important factor in preventing anxiety and depression. This chemical is found in the central nervous system, blood cells and the gastrointestinal tract, and is a regulator of mood, sleep and appetite.

The Amino Acid Tryptophan

To create serotonin, our body utilizes an amino acid called tryptophan, obtained from high protein foods. Tryptophan, from the protein we eat, is converted into serotonin, melatonin and vitamin B6 by the brain.

Our body cannot make its own tryptophan. Consuming food rich in protein is the only way our body has of obtaining this important amino acid.

Many IBS sufferers have been found to have unusually sensitive intestines and bowels. Because of this, diet has been suggested as a possible contributor to the severity of the symptoms.

However, as no particular food or food allergy has been found, it is not considered to be a factor in the onset of the condition.

Long Term Prognosis

There is no determined link between irritable bowel syndrome and the more serious bowel disorders, such as colitis and bowel cancer. Nevertheless, the symptoms are often painful and disruptive. It can be unpleasant, embarrassing and cause major trauma to the sufferers. It is a long-term problem that has a detrimental effect on the quality of life.

Symptoms of Irritable Bowel Syndrome (IBS)

The symptoms of irritable bowel syndrome vary from person to person. It is believed that one in five people experience some of the unpleasant symptoms of IBS at some time. Women are twice as likely to develop the condition as men. IBS rarely produces first time symptoms in people over forty.

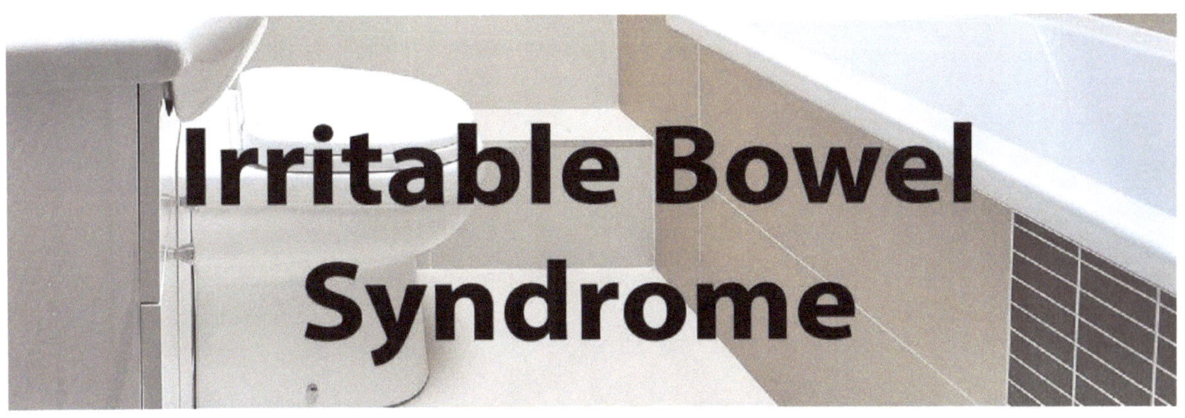

What is Irritable Bowel Syndrome (IBS)?

IBS is a gastrointestinal disorder. It is mainly characterized by several signs and symptoms that may include food intolerance, increased gas, bloating, indigestion and altered bowel habits. Those who suffer with IBS can also experience constipation, diarrhea, difficulty sleeping and fatigue.

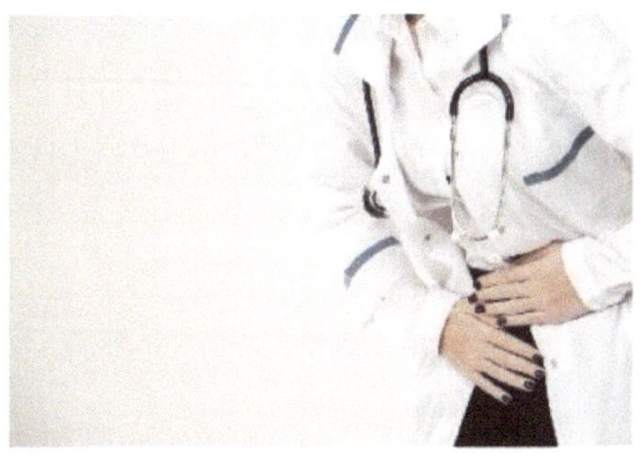

THERE ARE MANY PAINFUL AND EMBARRASSING SYMPTOMS OF IBS!

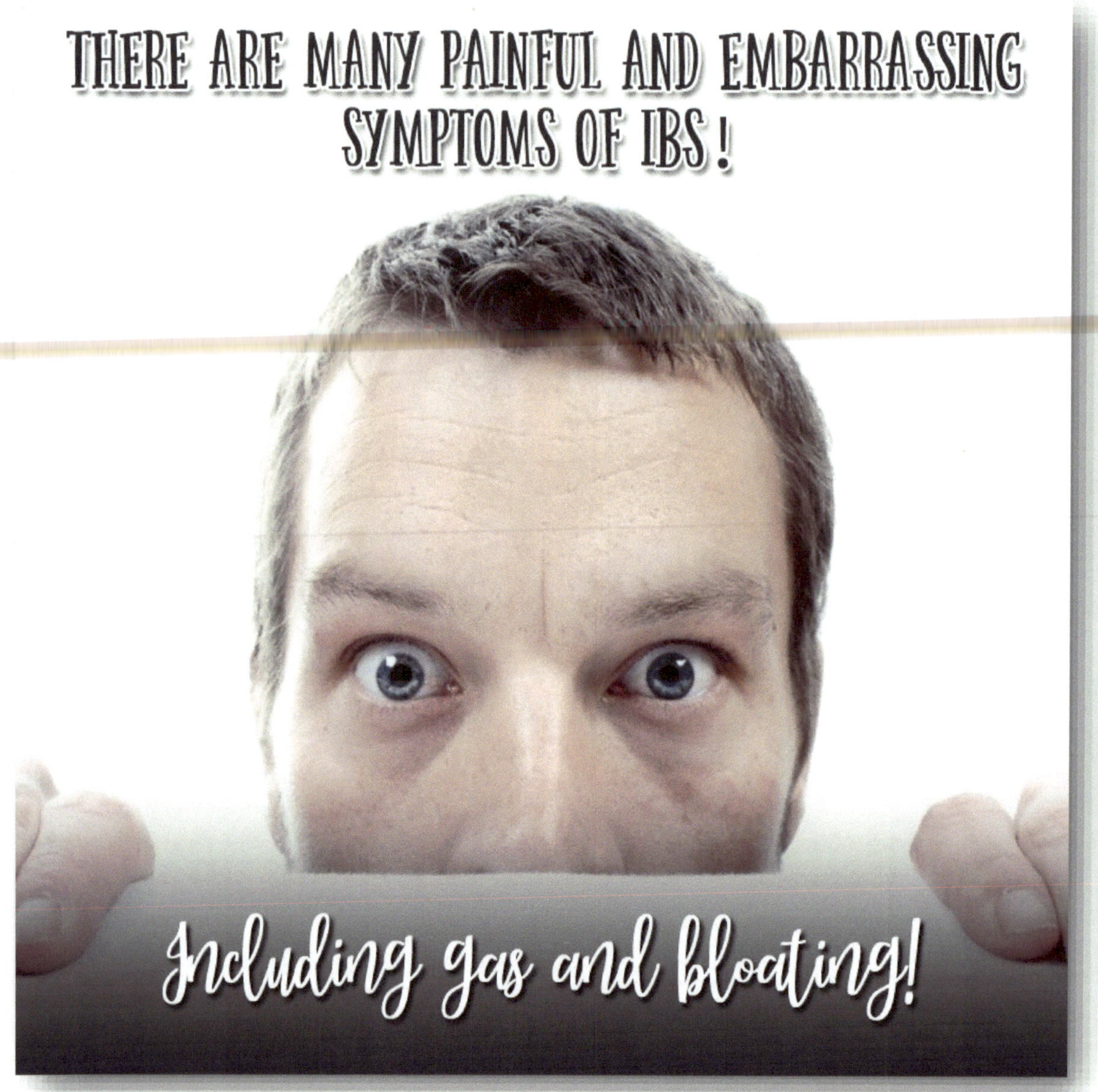

Some of these symptoms include diarrhea, constipation, abdominal pain, cramps, bloating, nausea, and vomiting. Diagnosis of IBS is difficult as none of these symptoms are restricted to this syndrome alone.

Diarrhea

Diarrhea is by far the most common symptom of IBS. However, it is interesting to note that in almost half of the known cases of IBS it does not cause diarrhea. If an attack of diarrhea is imminent the need to empty the bowels can be very persistent. When taken unaware in this situation the discomfort and embarrassment can be incredibly traumatic to the sufferer. Fear of these situations often results in people avoiding social situations.

A recent study involving 200 adults found that 12 bowel movements a week was the average for diarrhea-predominate IBS sufferers. This was more than twice the number of movements averaged by adult participants without IBS.

Constipation

More than 50% of IBS sufferers are constipation-predominate. Constipation is described as having less than three bowel movements per week. A symptom of IBS is the change in bowel movement. This change increases the speed of or slows down the regular transit of stool.

When the process slows, the bowel absorbs more water from the stool. This dries and hardens the stool, making it difficult to pass. Constipation-predominates often describes a sensation of incomplete bowel movement that encourages unnecessary straining.

Mixed or Alternating Diarrhea and Constipation

Mixed or alternating diarrhea and constipation affects approximately 20% of patients. This condition in people with IBS involves chronic recurring abdominal pain. The chronic pain component is the best clue that the condition is indeed IBS related, and not due to diet or other factors. This particular form of IBS is considered more severe than the others. The symptoms are more intense, and they tend to occur more frequently.

The sufferers of this mixed IBS also have more varying symptoms from one person to another, which requires the treatment to be more specific to each person's individual needs.

Pain and Cramping

Pain and cramping are also symptoms that is very common for people with irritable bowel syndrome. Researchers believe that when IBS is present the signals sent by the gut to the brain become distorted. This results in uncoordinated digestive tract muscles becoming tense and painful.

The pain can spread over a wide area of the abdomen. However, it can localize in the lower left area of the abdomen and tends to decrease following a bowel movement.

Gas and Bloating

Increased production of gas in the gut is the result of altered digestion caused by IBS. This in turn produces the uncomfortable feeling of bloating. Many patients claim that gas and bloating are the most persistent and irritating symptom of the condition.

Fatigue and Insomnia

Many studies have found that people with IBS often exhibit symptoms similar to insomniacs. They have difficulty getting to sleep and wake up feeling unrested. Over half of patients polled report low stamina and fatigue that affects the quality of their life.

Anxiety and Depression

A large study of 94,000 people found that men and women with IBS were 50% more likely to have an anxiety disorder. Over 70% were more likely to have a mood disorder such as depression than people who do not suffer from IBS.

The question of anxiety and depression is an unclear but vicious circle. Are IBS symptoms a result of mental stress, or does the stress of being an IBS sufferer make people more likely to suffer psychological problems?

Do You Know the Difference Between Irritable Bowel Syndrome (IBS) or Inflammatory Bowel Disorder (IBD)?

Both chronic gastrointestinal conditions have similar names and share some similar symptoms.

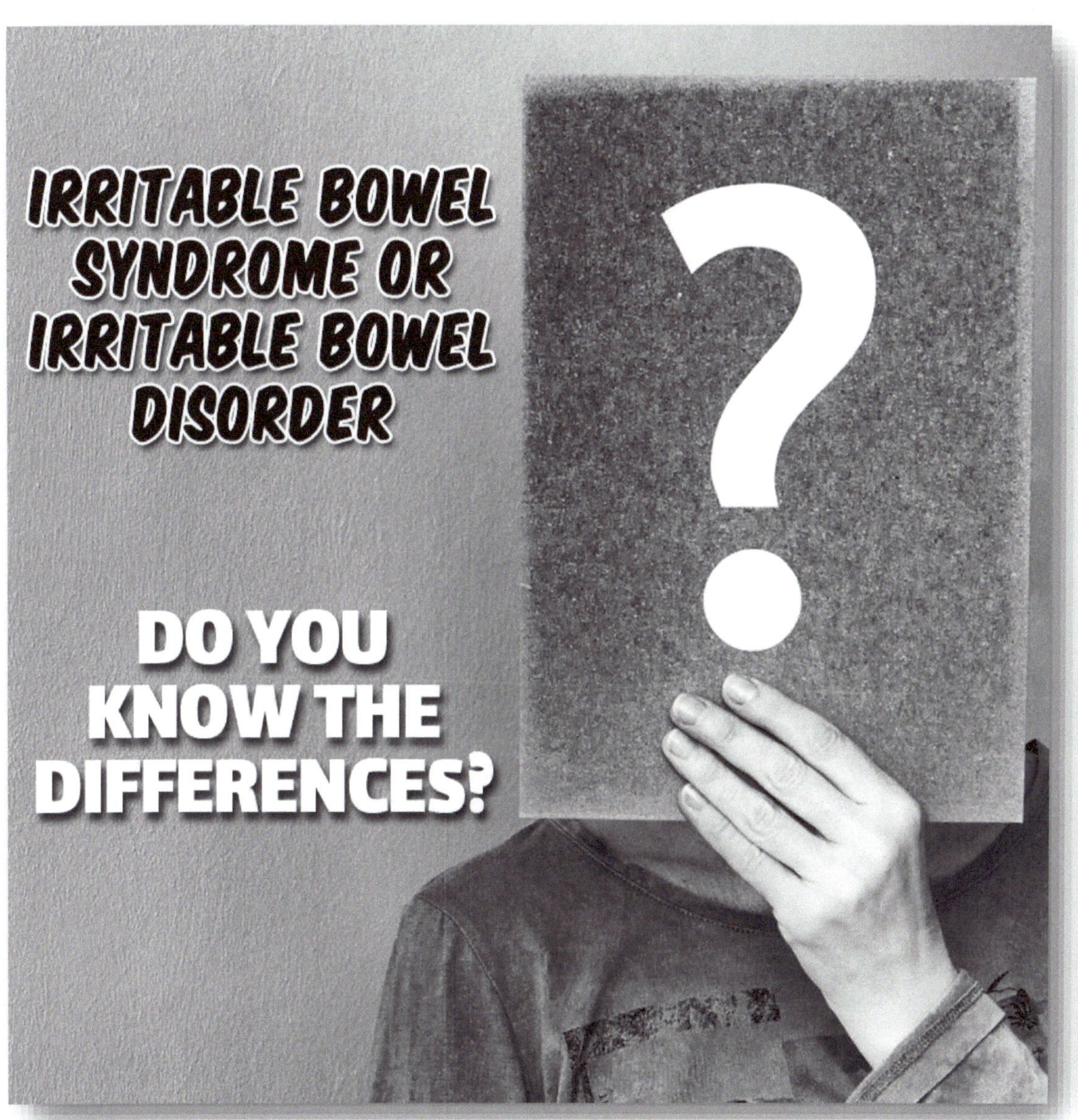

Symptoms Common to Both Disorders

Abdominal pain, diarrhea, abdominal cramping, nausea, vomiting, and the urgent need for bowel elimination are all common symptoms of both IBS and IBD.

However, both of these conditions have symptoms that are distinctly different from each other. Inflammatory bowel disorder is the more serious of the two conditions.

What Causes Irritable Bowel Syndrome (IBS)?

Irritable bowel syndrome is classified as a functional disorder, not a disease. This classification means the symptoms have no identifiable cause. Other conditions in the functional disorder category are chronic fatigue syndrome and tension headaches.

The causes of IBS are speculative and indicate that the symptoms begin because of faulty communication between the nervous system and the muscles of the bowel. Other researchers have suggested food or stress may trigger symptoms.

Symptoms Unique to Irritable Bowel Syndrome

One distinct symptom is changes in bowel movements, involving alternate bouts of diarrhea and constipation. These changes are determined by the speed it takes the stool to transit from the colon to the rectum.

Other symptoms not relevant to IBD are stools containing whitish mucus, a sensation of not having a complete evacuation during bowel movements and abdominal bloating.

IBS is a common functional disorder involving the colon. It does not have complications that lead to any other more serious bowel related conditions. However, it does have minor complications that sufferers of IBS need to be aware of.

Dehydration

Continual severe diarrhea over a long period can cause the body to lose so much water and salt that you can become dehydrated. Patients suffering from diarrhea-predominant IBS should be aware of this and increase their intake of fluids, especially water.

Impacted Bowel

Long-term constipation can cause the stool to become so hard that it gets blocked in the colon. This is known as fecal impaction and it can be painful and cause headaches, nausea and vomiting. Patients with constipation-predominant IBS are most at risk, and it more prevalent in older people.

Treatment for IBS

Symptoms of mild cases of IBS can often be controlled by good management of diet and stress. Appropriate lifestyle changes can also be beneficial in both areas.

For people with more severe symptoms, counseling and/or medication may be needed. This is sometimes the recommendation when the symptoms involve severe stress and depression.

Many medical professionals are recommending the FODMAPs diet as the first line of treatment for irritable bowel syndrome.

What Causes Inflammatory Bowel Disorder (IBD)?

The exact cause of IBD is not known. Researchers believe that the IBD types, Crohn's disease and ulcerative colitis, are the result of an immune system error that causes inflammation to bowel tissue. It is believed that sufferers of these conditions have a genetic predisposition to IBD.

Symptoms Unique to Inflammatory Bowel Disorder

IBD is a much more serious disease than IBS. Crohn's disease and ulcerative colitis are the two most serious disorders from a group of diseases involving inflammation of the digestive tract.

IBD causes tissue to become ulcerated in the digestive tract. These ulcers can appear anywhere along the digestive tract from the mouth to the anus.

Any part of the gastrointestinal tract can be affected by Crohn's disease. The large and small intestines, anus and rectum are all areas of the body that are affected by ulcerative colitis.

Other symptoms of IBD are rectal bleeding, anemia, pain and redness of the eyes, fever, joint pain, no appetite, weight loss and tiredness.

IBD requires a more intense treatment regimen than IBS. Patients have a much higher risk of serious of long-term complications.

Treatment for IBD

The predominant aim in the treatment of IBD is to reduce inflammation. Reduced inflammation can relieve the symptoms that lead to complications. The best-case scenario is long-term remission. This condition requires drug therapy and sometimes surgery.

Could It Be Colon Cancer Instead?

During the process of diagnosing an individual for IBS, additional tests must be performed to rule out any possibility of colon cancer. This is important as there have been some cases where colon cancer was incorrectly diagnosed as IBS. Naturally, this means that a misdiagnosis causes the patient to not promptly receive the right treatment for their condition.

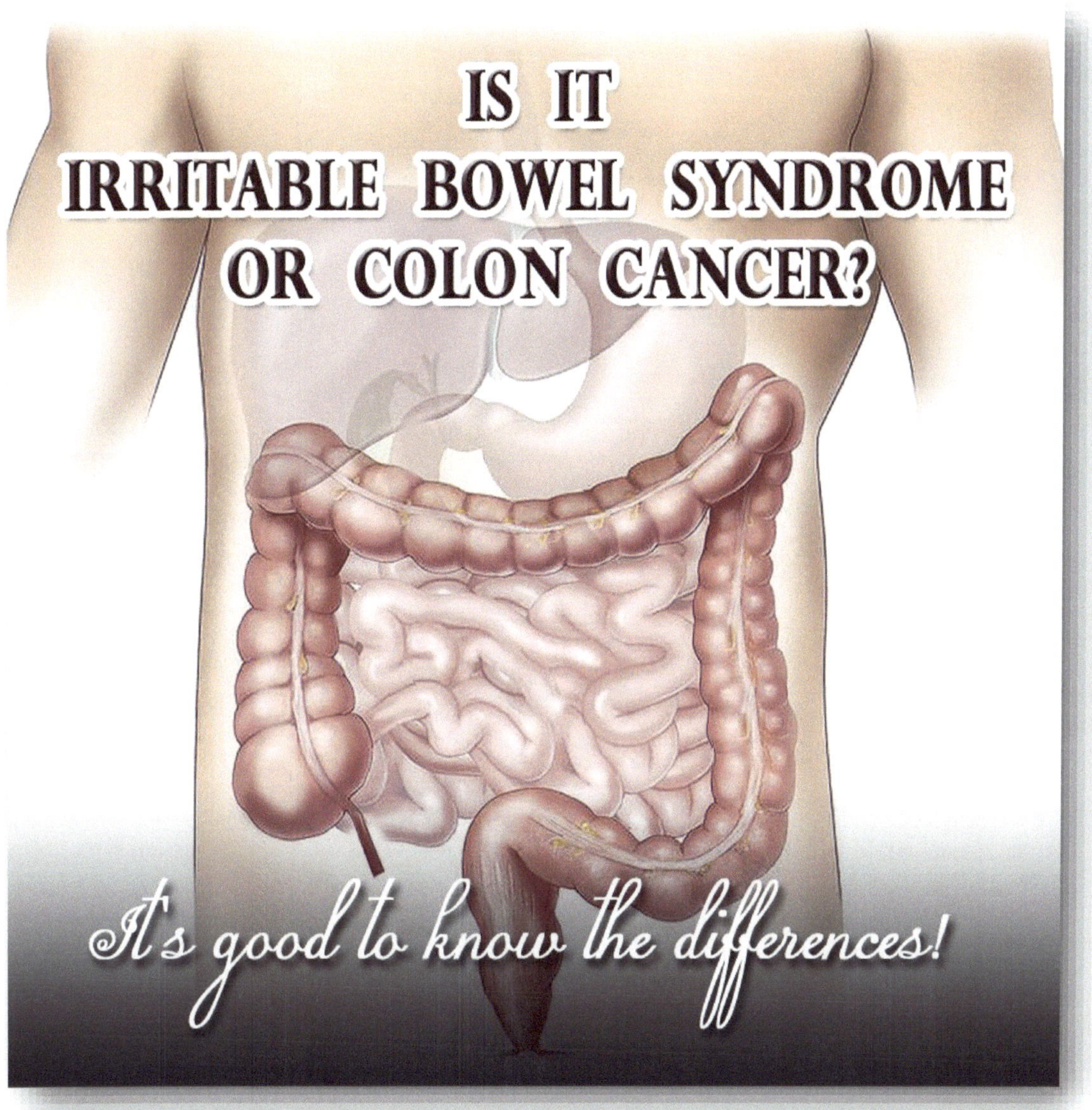

Colon cancer occurs because of abnormal cells growing in the colon. Once these cancerous cells multiply in the colon wall, cancer can spread to other parts of the body. Colon cancer patients are often initially diagnosed due to a cancerous lump in their rectum or stomach.

IBS is a functional disorder that mainly affects the digestive tract. Those who have IBS are less likely to have detectable abnormalities in their digestive system, yet they exhibit symptoms that can be painful, distressing and very troublesome.

To date, there isn't any conclusive evidence to prove the exact cause behind the emergence of IBS symptoms. This is the reason why there aren't any specific tests for diagnosing IBS. However, many experts believe that food intolerances, bacteria overgrowth, stress and an unhealthy lifestyle may all play a part in triggering IBS symptoms.

Differences and Similarities between IBS and Colon Cancer Symptoms

People who have IBS or colon cancer may find themselves feeling the "urge" to go to the toilet, even though they've just finished a bowel movement.

One distinct symptom that colon cancer may exhibit, and IBS does not, is rectal bleeding. However, if you do see blood in your stool, do not immediately jump to the conclusion that you have colon cancer. Some people experience blood in their stools which is caused by other conditions, including hemorrhoids.

Another possible sign that it could be colon cancer, is that the patient may appear to be anemic and have rectal pain. Colon cancer increases a person's risk of suffering from unintentional weight loss.

On the other hand, IBS sufferers may experience bloating, stomach pain and abdominal cramps, and release mucus from their rectum. Another problem is experiencing bouts of diarrhea and constipation. These issues are common among IBS sufferers.

Frequently experiencing intestinal gas, which adds to abdominal discomfort, can also be experienced by people with IBS. Tension or a feeling of hardness in the stomach right after eating is yet another symptom of IBS.

Alarming Symptoms to Watch Out For

Here are some warning symptoms that are not brought on by IBS. In most cases, these symptoms occur because of a serious disease, such as cancer, or another co-occurring condition. You should consult your doctor immediately if you experience the following:

- You have specific symptoms that occur only at night.
- You are losing weight and have no idea why.
- You are seeing blood in your stools.

Some cases of colon cancer start out as being benign but may later develop into being cancerous. Individuals with a benign tumor must be extra vigilant about any changes in their health. These people are more at risk:

- People who are aged 60 and above.
- People who regularly eat processed foods and red meat.
- Individuals diagnosed or who have a family history of Crohn's disease, celiac disease, inflammatory bowel disease and/or ulcerative colitis.
- People who smoke and drink alcohol to excess.

Diagnosing IBS and Colon Cancer

IBS is most likely given as a diagnosis after ruling out the possibility of any other conditions such as cancer, infection or celiac disease. Although IBS symptoms cause discomfort and can be very distressing, it does not increase your risk for other conditions such as Crohn's disease, ulcerative colitis or cancer.

If colon cancer is detected early, the chances of a successful outcome is increased. Screening for colon cancer may include blood tests and biopsy analysis. The colon will be examined via a colonoscopy, sigmoidoscopy, stool DNA test, or a combination of these. If you have any digestive problems, be proactive and ask your doctor to perform some tests for you. IBS symptoms are distressing enough, but do not be complacent about ensuring that these symptoms are not masking something more serious.

IBS, Celiac Disease, and Crohn's Disease Oh My!

Digestive problems are common; however, you don't hear people discussing them as quickly as they do the windy weather. Let's face it, not many people want to discuss their 'windy' flatulence problem. Therefore, many people suffer in silence.

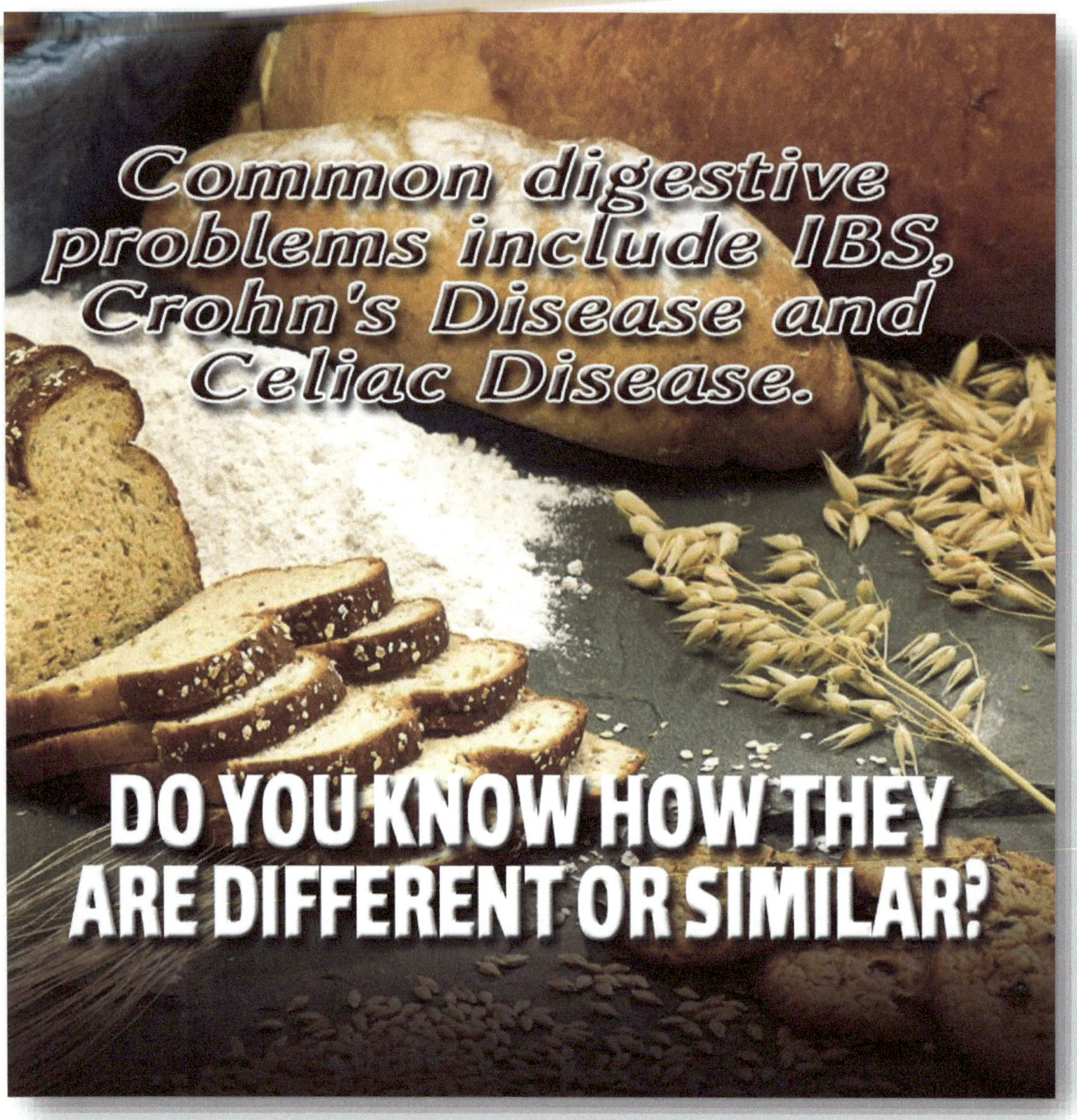

This is another reason why so many people who have digestive problems are still undiagnosed. They simple don't realize they may have more than a little problem.

Some of the most common digestive problems are IBS, Crohn's disease and Celiac disease. Let's look at how they may be different or similar.

Celiac Disease vs. IBS

Celiac Disease and IBS can cause diarrhea, bloating and gas. However, Celiac disease can also have other symptoms which manifest as joint pain, dental defects and osteoporosis. People who suffer from Celiac disease may also suffer from loss of bone density, fatigue, blistery skin, anemia, headaches, heartburn, impaired functioning of the spleen and nervous system injury.

If you do not have any symptoms of IBS, chances are you do not have IBS! However, in the case of Celiac disease, you can have this disease without showing any obvious symptoms. If you have IBS, your bowel movement is affected but this may not be so when you have Celiac disease. You *may* be sensitive to gluten when you are diagnosed with IBS, whereas gluten is usually the leading cause of celiac disease.

The Causes of Celiac Disease and IBS

To date, the exact cause of Celiac disease remains unknown. However, data from numerous studies have shown that when an individual with Celiac disease consumes gluten, his immune system attacks it as if it is a threat. This triggers the emergence of several other symptoms of Celiac disease.

Unfortunately, this attack by the immune system on the gluten not only causes unwanted symptoms, it also can lead to the gradual damage of the intestines, which makes this condition even more dangerous.

This is because damage to the intestines, specifically the villi, causes them to be much less efficient in absorbing nutrients from the food ingested. As a result, malnutrition becomes a highly increased risk.

Another possible cause of Celiac disease is gene mutation, which may arise after a person has had a viral infection, surgery or pregnancy.

Just like Celiac disease, the exact cause of IBS is also not yet known. Many experts have speculated that IBS symptoms arise due to several factors. Some of these include infections, gastrointestinal motility problems, pain sensitivity, small intestinal bacterial overgrowth and brain-gut signal problems.

Other factors that may also contribute to the occurrence of IBS symptoms include food sensitivities, neurotransmitters, mental health issues and genetics.

The Co-Occurrence of Celiac Disease and IBS

A 2014 study suggests that there could be links between IBS and celiac disease. Experts made an assessment on 992 children who were diagnosed with IBS, functional abdominal pain and dyspepsia. The results of their blood tests revealed that 15% of the children had celiac disease and from this same group of children researchers found that 12% of them were also suffering from IBS.

Data from this study led doctors to suggest that laboratory screening for children with celiac disease should be extended. By doing this, doctors will be able to determine whether there is a co-occurrence of these two digestive problems.

The Prevalence of Celiac Disease and IBS

In the United States alone, one out of 133 people have been found to be suffering from Celiac Disease. This condition has been found to be more prevalent in men than in women. Unfortunately, 83% of sufferers were previously undiagnosed or misdiagnosed. This shows that the possibility of Celiac Disease could be even higher.

This condition is also more common among Type 1 diabetics, people with Turner syndrome, Down syndrome, collagenous colitis or autoimmune disease. People whose first-degree relatives are suffering from Celiac disease also face a higher risk of developing the condition.

Alternatively, IBS is found to be more prevalent in women rather than men. This is also the most common gastrointestinal condition, according to gastroenterologists. It accounts for an estimated $21 billion of lost productivity in the workplace.

Crohn's Disease vs. IBS

Crohn's disease is an autoimmune condition. People with Crohn's disease suffer from an autoimmune attack from their mouth to their anus. This leads to very painful inflammation as well as intestinal ulcers.

Those who are diagnosed with Crohn's disease may also experience fever and blood loss. People diagnosed with IBS will find themselves passing large amounts of mucus, while those with Crohn's disease will excrete only a small amount of mucus, and this can affect the process of eliminating waste.

Crohn's disease patients also face a higher risk of developing a skin condition called psoriasis, while those with IBS may not have it at all.

Crohn's Disease vs. Celiac Disease

Celiac and Crohn's disease have many things in common. They have plenty of similarities both symptomatic and genetic. However, there are important differences between the two.

Some of the symptoms that are common to both include anemia, diarrhea, fever, abdominal pain, rectal bleeding, weight loss and intestinal inflammation. Results from studies conducted have revealed that Crohn's disease and Celiac disease both have a genetic influence. Those who have Celiac disease are also at risk of having Crohn's disease.

Sufferers of Crohn's disease may experience fever, diarrhea, mouth sores, weight loss and abdominal pain. They may also see some blood in their stools and have perianal disease.

Sufferers of Celiac disease may experience vomiting, abdominal pain and bloating. They are more likely to experience diarrhea and/or constipation. Their stools are usually fatty, foul-smelling and pale in color.

The Anxiety and Stress Factor

Almost 60% of people diagnosed with IBS have been found to be suffering from a psychiatric disorder. This is according to Edward Blanchard, a psychology professor.

He added that the most common type of anxiety that people with IBS exhibit is GAD - Generalized Anxiety Disorder, while 20% of these IBS sufferers also had

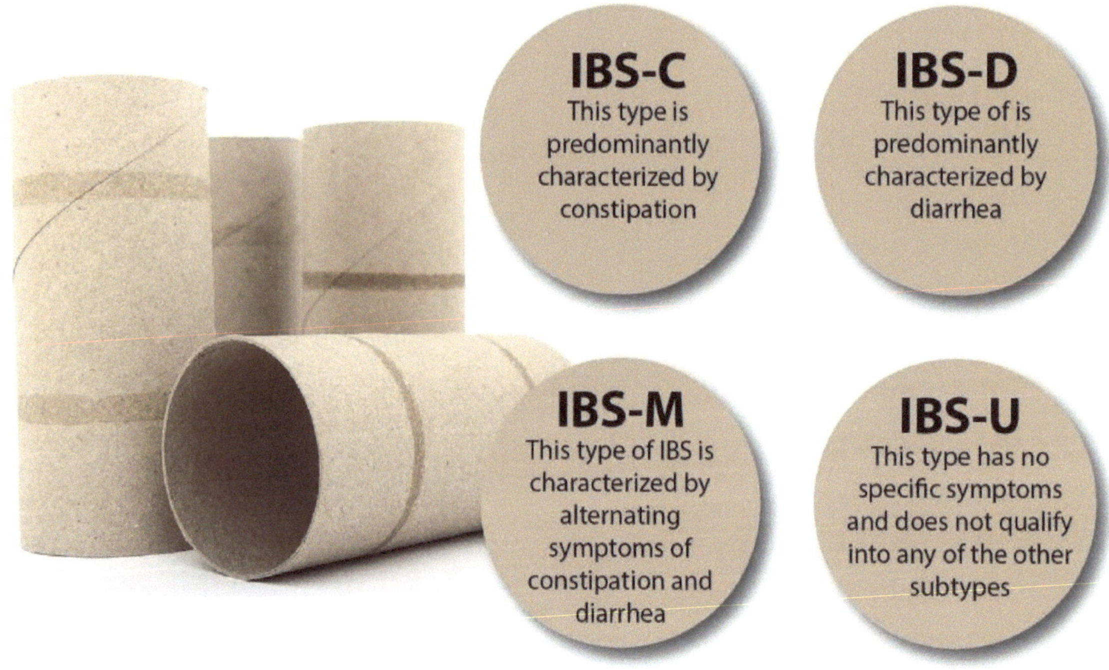

depression.

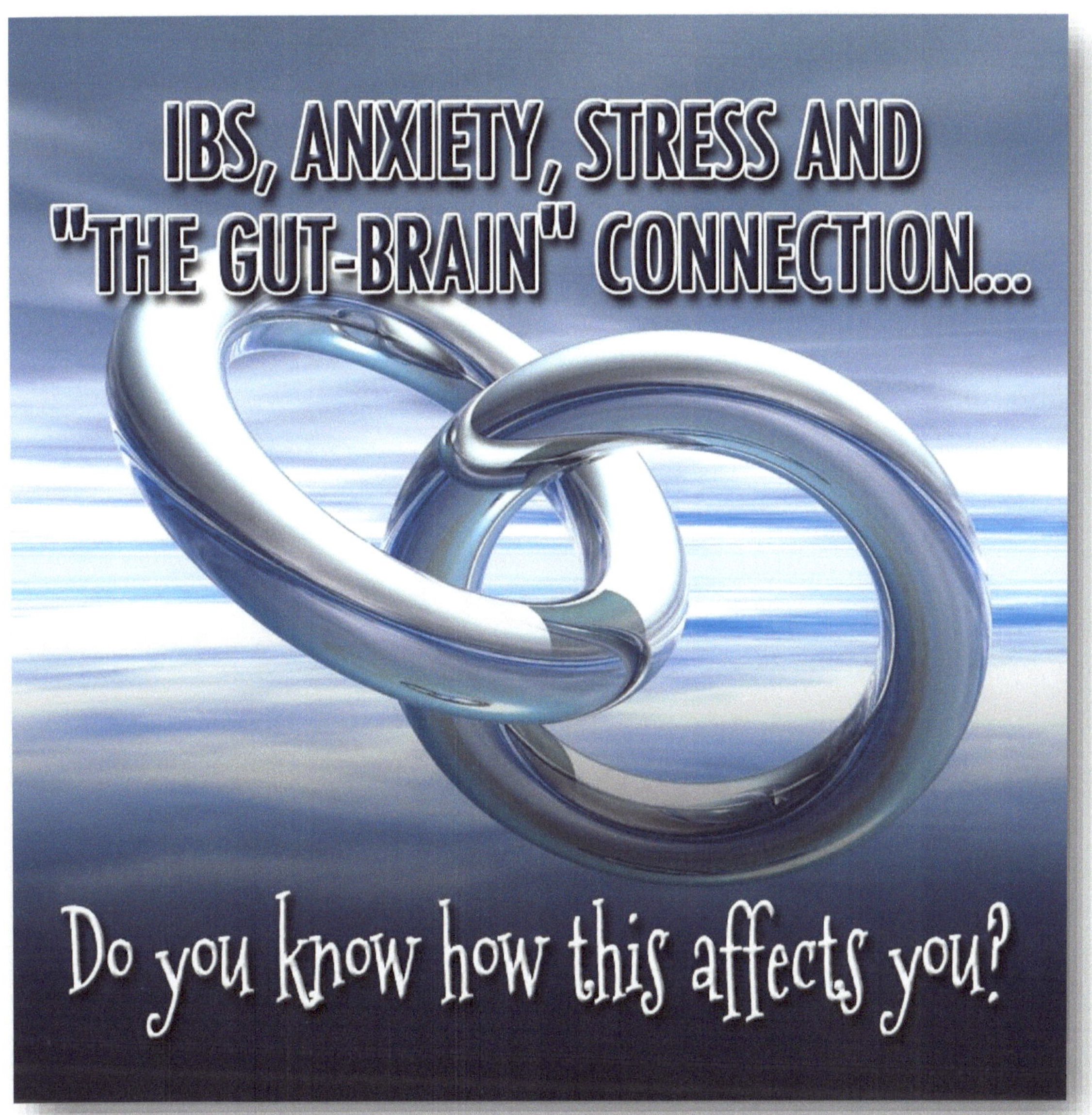

The Gut-Brain Connection

Have you heard about the gut being the second brain? If you haven't, the human gut is made up of a network of neurons that are very complex. This network is referred to as the gut's brain which is hardwired to the brain in your head.

This significant link between the brain and the gut is what we call the gut-brain axis. They're working like a two-way street. The brain sends signals to the gut while the gut can send signals to the brain.

Needless to say, your brain influences your gut function and your gut can affect your brain functioning. The concept of the gut affecting brain functions and vice versa is not considered as being "new information".

In the early 20th century, crude experiments that were conducted showed that by making alterations to the person's emotional state, their blood flow was affected.

In addition, this alteration in emotional state had an impact on the proper flow of food and waste from the gut and out of the body. A modern field of research referred to as neurogastroenterology has scientific proof that shows how the brain and the gut interact with each other.

The Link Between Stress, Anxiety and IBS

Numerous experiments have shown that people with IBS have been found to have a stronger gastrointestinal reaction to any stressful situation compared to individuals who do not have IBS.

Experiencing stress and other strong emotional reactions may trigger intestinal motility problems among people with IBS, compared to those who do not have IBS. This is because IBS increases visceral sensitivity, which is characterized by an intense feeling of pain in the internal organs. Conversely stress has been found to worsen visceral sensitivity.

Stress is known to increase permeability of the intestinal wall. This translates to the increased likelihood of harmful bacteria and food particles entering the bloodstream. Unfortunately, this occurrence opens more risks for developing gut problems and other health issues.

Pain and discomfort responses to bowel inflammation and other problems associated with increased motility will also quickly reach the brain. Remember, the gut and the brain have a special channel for passing information quickly.

Once these signals are sent to the brain, greater levels of pain are experienced, thereby adding to the development of anxiety and stress. Many experts believe that anxiety is one of the main causes of Irritable Bowel Syndrome.

However, not all people with anxiety are suffering from the symptoms of IBS. Some experts say it can be caused by having low levels of neurotransmitters, such as serotonin, and in turn the gut senses this and triggers IBS symptoms.

Aside from stress and anxiety, IBS is common in people who have psychological problems such as depression, post-traumatic stress disorder or PTSD, Obsessive-Compulsive Disorder or OCD and panic disorder.

Heal Your Irritable Bowel Syndrome (IBS) The Natural Way

Many IBS sufferers have already tried pharmaceutical drugs and other medical treatments recommended by their doctor. Many of these patients would have had little or no success with these treatments.

Alternate Health Care Treatments

Natural therapies have proven very beneficial in the treatment of many illnesses, including IBS. Here are a few that have given relief to many sufferers.

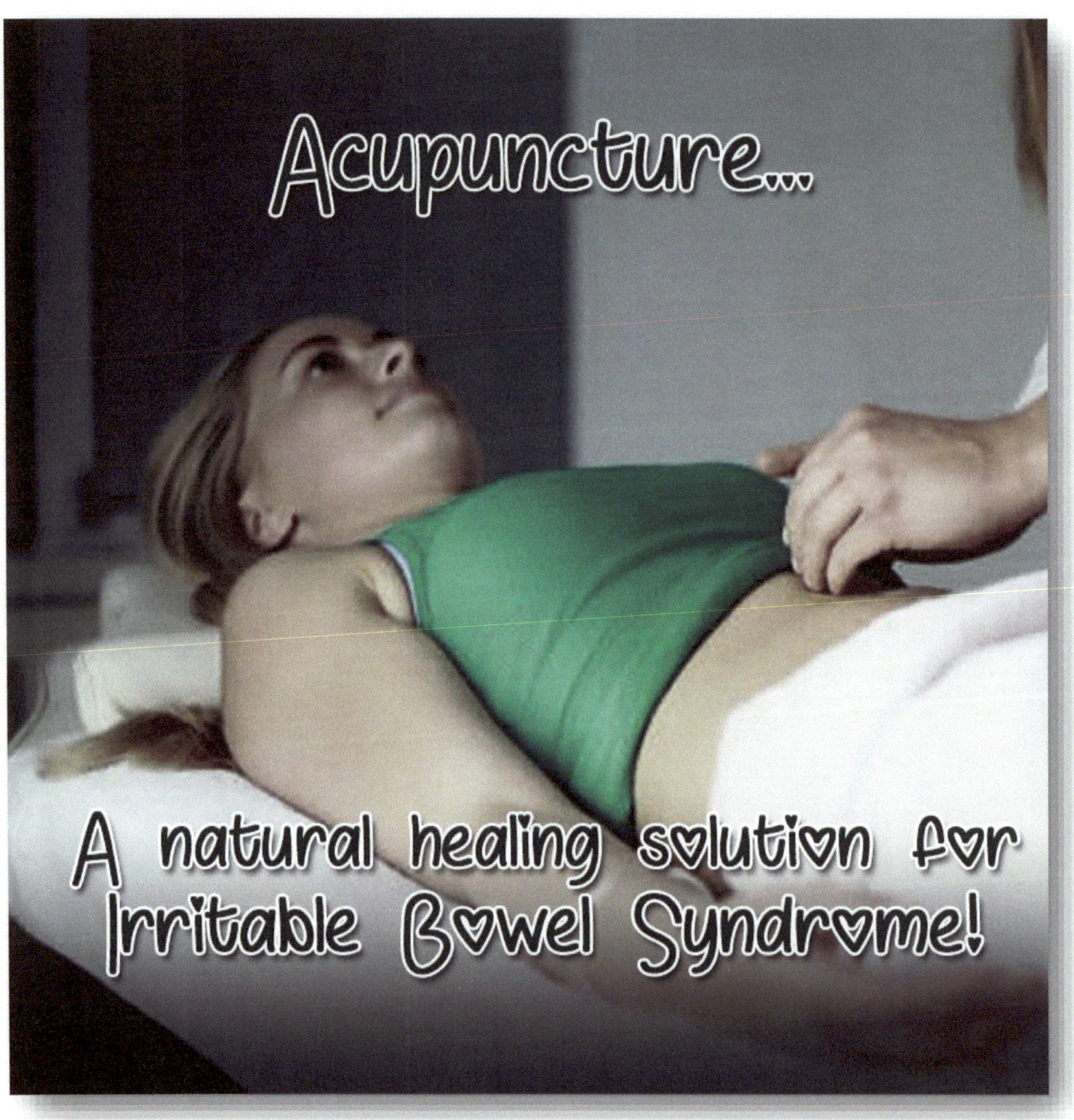

Acupuncture

Acupuncture is a beneficial therapy for chronic pain. It is not fully understood how this traditional Chinese treatment works. Masters of this therapy believe the needles stimulate electronic signals in the body.

They explain that the signals either encourage the body to release pain killing chemicals, or they activate the body's natural healing system. Acupuncture is a popular alternative therapy for IBS; some tests have found it to be very helpful in the relief of stomach pain and bloating.

Hypnosis

Many studies have been conducted to determine if focusing the mind with hypnotherapy is able to improve the emotional and physical symptoms in people with IBS.

Results of these studies have been very encouraging. Study sessions that have focused on the problems the participants had with IBS have led to long term improvement in both emotional and physical health. Follow-up research found the improvement had been maintained six months after the studies had ended.

Cognitive Behavior Therapy (CBT)

Cognitive behavior therapy teaches people to identify and change false opinions they have formed about themselves over the years. It is used to train people with IBS how they can ease their symptoms and improve their quality of life.

In a study, researchers gave a group of IBS patients up to 10 weeks CBT therapy sessions. The sessions covered information on IBS, and muscle relaxation training. Sessions on ways to curb worries about the illness were included.

The patients were also taught how to develop a flexible set of problem-solving skills related to IBS. Results showed that 60% to75% of participants had improvement in their symptoms.

Probiotics

Probiotics are live bacteria found in fermented food like yogurt, kefir and is also available in supplements. Several published reviews on random clinical trials included problotics and placebos in a study. Probiotics proved to have a better result in relieving abdominal pain and other IBS symptoms than placebos.

IBS is a disorder characterized by abdominal pain, diarrhea or constipation, or a combination of both. Symptoms vary from patient to patient, so it is understandable that what provides relief for one person, will not necessarily work for another.

Some alternate health professionals believe probiotics are very worthwhile. They are known to restore the good bacteria in the gut. An added benefit is that studies have shown that they do not appear to have any side effects.

Supplements

As well as probiotics, supplements such as evening primrose oil, borage oil and fish oil may also be helpful in relieving symptoms of IBS. The oil supplements are known to have a calming effect on the gut. Primrose oil supplements are especially helpful to women during their menstrual cycle. Many have found primrose oil relieves pain, discomfort and bloating, that can increase at this time of the month.

Herbs

Some herbs have found favor with a lot of IBS sufferers. Peppermint and ginger have been shown to have a calming effect on the muscles of the colon. When the muscles in the colon are tense, symptoms like diarrhea and abdominal discomfort increase. This is why peppermint and ginger tea is popular with IBS patients.

Herbs and supplements may react adversely with some medications. It is advisable to talk to your doctor or pharmacist if you are taking any prescribed medication.

Probiotics for IBS

Bacteria inside our gut serves as important determinant of any disease present or alternatively, the status of our overall health. If the population of beneficial bacteria is not kept in balance, a person becomes vulnerable to many different types of gut problems. Increasing research indicates that a wide range of human health problems are caused or exacerbated by poor gut health.

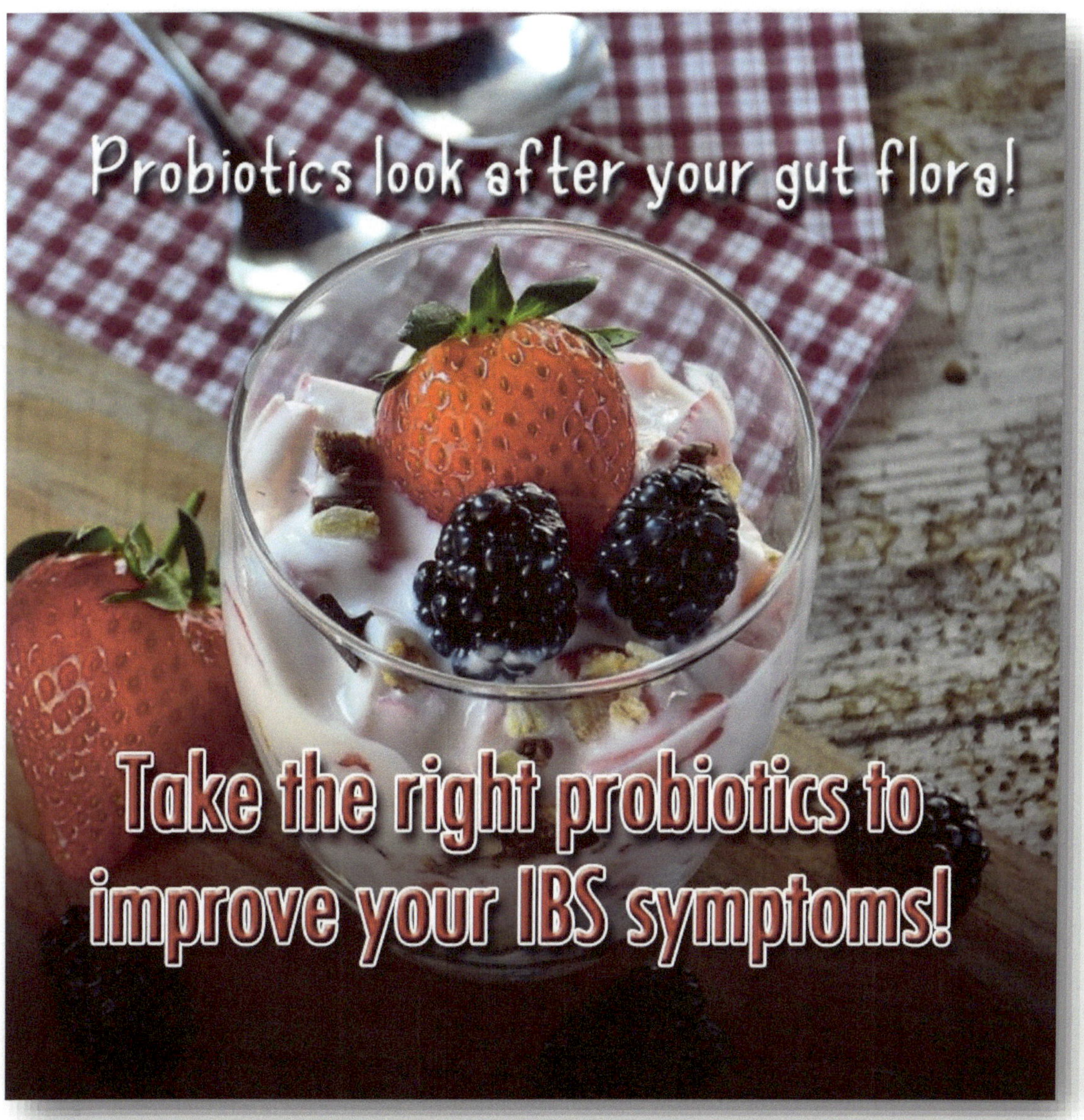

If the population of these beneficial bacteria, also known as gut flora, becomes unbalanced, harmful bacteria can take over and outnumber the good bacteria. If this happens it can allow the gut to become an ideal breeding place for disease. It can also cause painful IBS symptoms.

One of the best-known ways to prevent or remedy this situation is to take probiotics on a daily basis.

What are Probiotics?

Probiotics are live microorganisms that can be obtained from specific foods or supplements. When consumed correctly, these probiotics can help boost your health and fight against disease.

Some excellent food sources of probiotics are sauerkraut, kimchi, yogurt and tempeh. The most common types of probiotics that are obtained from foods and supplements are Bifidobacterium and Lactobacillus.

Probiotics and Its Impact on IBS Sufferers

Experts have discovered that IBS sufferers do not have enough Bifidobacterium and Lactobacillus in their gut. Instead, IBS sufferers have higher levels of harmful bacteria, such as Clostridium, Streptococcus and E. coli.

Studies have revealed that the small intestines of almost 85% of IBS sufferers had harmful bacterial overgrowth. This overgrowth triggers the emergence of several symptoms. However, whether this bacterial overgrowth is the result of IBS or it's the problem causing it, remains to be seen.

Changes in the population ratios of bacteria in the gut can trigger the symptoms of IBS as it promotes inflammation and increases gas sensitivity in the intestines. An imbalanced gut flora can greatly reduce the ability of the immune system to fight against disease, while also affecting its digestive motility.

How Probiotics Can Help IBS Sufferers

A study funded by the National Institutes of Health indicated that probiotics can help improve IBS symptoms by preventing the continuous growth of disease-causing bacteria in the gut.

These probiotics have been found to improve the barrier functions of the immune system. Regular consumption of probiotics has led to the reduction of the gut's sensitivity to gas while also improving the gut's ability to fight inflammation.

Probiotics boost the population of healthy bacteria in the gut and helps restore proper gut flora balance. This reduces the non-beneficial bacterial populations to natural and non-injurious levels. Healthy ratios prevent excessive gas production and other symptoms of digestive discomforts, including IBS.

Probiotics assist in breaking down foods that can trigger IBS symptoms. The healthy bacteria also help modulate the enteric nervous system (i.e. the gut's nervous system) and this largely reduces the adverse impact of stress in the gut, making it ideal for people with stress-induced IBS.

Here is a list of probiotic strains that are beneficial for IBS Sufferers:

- Lactococcus lactis Rosell 1058
- Lactobacillus plantarum 299v
- Bifidobacterium lactis
- Bifidobacterium infantis 35624
- Bifidobacterium bifidum MIMBb75
- Lactobacillus rhamnosus GG
- Lactobacillus brevis

It is necessary to be aware that not all probiotics are the same. They do vary in types and which bacterial populations they benefit, therefore how they affect an individual may vary.

It is also important to note that the benefits of taking probiotics are not experienced immediately. It may take a few weeks before any effects are experienced as the beneficial bacterial colonies increase.

Probiotics for IBS Sufferers

- **Bifidobacterium infantis**
  This bacteria has been found to be effective in relieving IBS symptoms such as bloating, bowel movement and abdominal pain.

- **Bifidobacterium bifidum**
  A clinical trial showed that almost 50 percent of study participants experienced improvement of IBS symptoms with this probiotic bacteria.

- **Bifidobacterium lactis**
  This probiotic bacteria is found beneficial in providing relief from stress-related IBS symptoms, which may include permeability and gut sensitivity.

- **Lactobacillus brevis**
  This reduces the frequency of diarrhea and abdominal pain.

- **Lactobacillus plantarum**
  This is helpful in relieving bloating and abdominal pain.

- **Lactobacillus rhamnosus GG**
  This bacteria helps reduce abdominal pain among children with IBS.

- **Bacillus coagulans**
  This is beneficial in providing relief from bloating and abdominal pain.

Alternatively, if you notice your symptoms getting worse while consuming probiotics, stop taking them immediately and consult your doctor.

Effective Yoga Poses for Irritable Bowel Syndrome Relief

IBS or Irritable Bowel Syndrome is a functional bowel disorder characterized by erratic bowel movements, such as diarrhea and constipation. If you suffer from symptoms that cause discomfort, there are several natural, non-invasive ways to reduce the intensity, duration and frequency of your IBS symptoms.

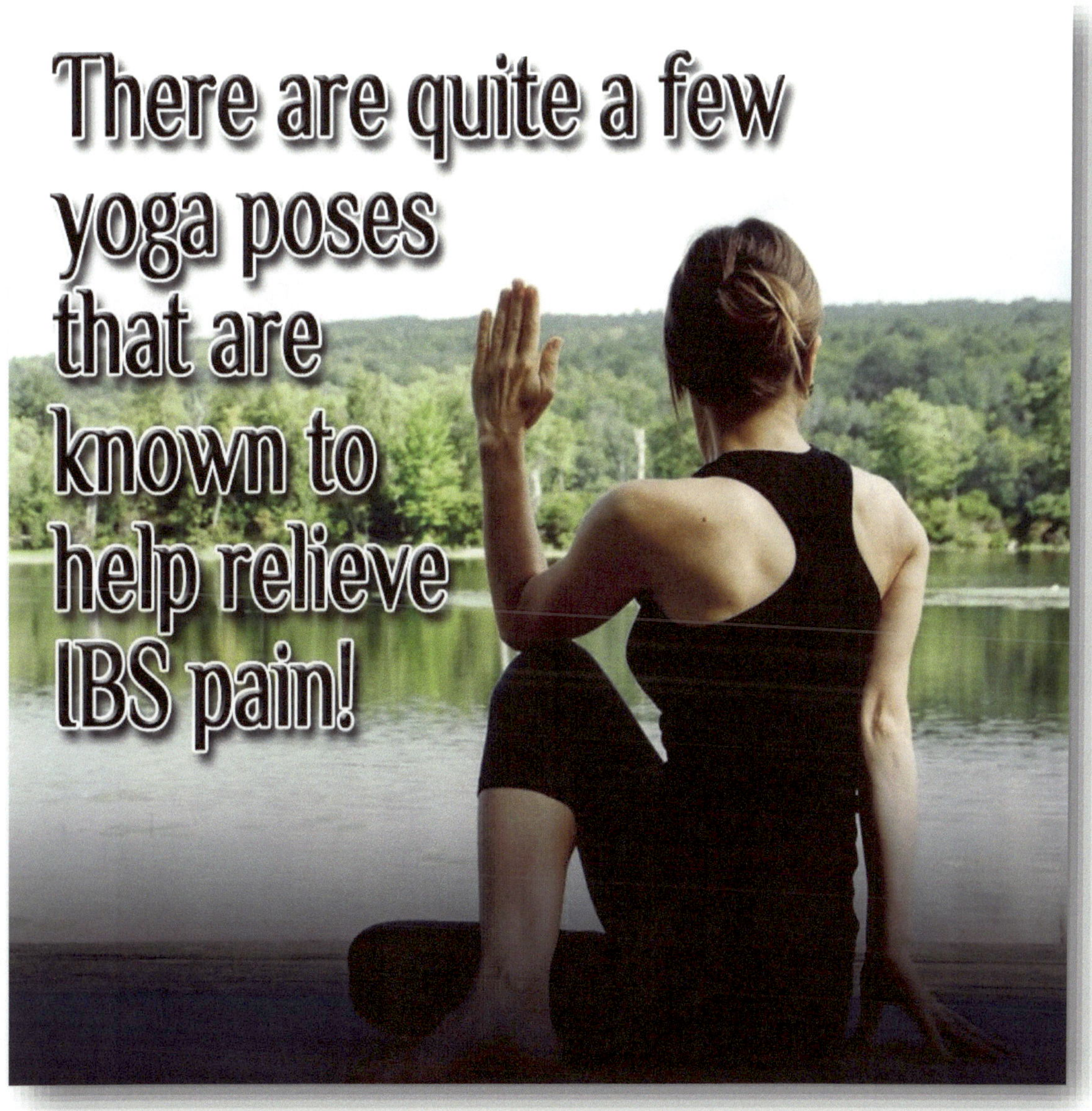

There appear to be a strong link between stress and anxiety, and the incidence of IBS symptoms. Chronic exposure to stress can trigger or worsen IBS symptoms, therefore, preventing or alleviating IBS effects should extend beyond dietary adjustments.

For a multitude of reasons, including reducing IBS symptoms, it is highly beneficial to lower your stress levels. One of the best ways to do this is through yoga. Here are a few yoga poses that are known to help relieve IBS pain and discomfort.

Parighasana (Gate Pose)

This pose allows the sides of your torso to be stretched and your internal organs to be stimulated. Parighasana pose will improve your breathing and lung capacity while also aiding in your digestion. Your core strength is also developed as it improves your body's ability to eliminate waste.

Ardha Matsyendrasana (Half-Seated Spinal Twist)

This pose allows more air to enter your lungs as it opens your chest. The increased levels of oxygen promote an improved ability to flush out excess toxins. This pose also stimulates your kidneys and improves your digestive functions. Performing this half-seated spinal twist pose on a regular basis will also help eliminate fatigue.

Ananda Balasana (Happy Baby Pose)

Happy Baby Pose is a great stress and pain reliever. It works effectively in soothing your spine and releasing tension in the back. For IBS sufferers, this pose compresses the stomach, and acts as an internal massage on your organs.

Dhanurasana (Bow Pose)

The Bow Pose not only helps relieve stress. It has been found helpful in relieving constipation and improves the functioning of your intestines and overall digestive system.

Pavanamuktasana (Wind Relieving Pose)

This wind relieving pose works to strengthen your abdominal muscles while
making it possible for the insides of your abdomen to be massaged.
It helps your body to release toxic gases, reduce acidity and provide relief from
constipation. Performing this yoga pose also releases tension in the neck and
lower back.

Bhujangasana (Cobra Pose)

This pose is good for stretching and toning the abdomen. It is helpful in
improving circulation and in fighting against the symptoms of stress and
fatigue.

Adho Mukha Svanasana (Downward Facing Dog)

This pose is beneficial in toning the abdominal muscles, stretching the spine
and improving digestion. This pose is helpful for boosting blood flow and
beneficial in calming the mind and boosting energy levels.

Make Yoga a Lifestyle Change

To gain maximum benefit from these yoga poses, perform them regularly. A
once-off session may provide some temporary relief, but to truly appreciate
the benefits, you need to incorporate them into your IBS treatment plan. They
need to be performed daily if possible.

Don't start too aggressively. Start slow, and if you need help, perform these
exercises under the supervision of an expert yoga instructor. Remember that
these poses put pressure on your body parts and internal organs.

Yoga can have a hugely positive impact on how you manage stress and
improve your attitude towards your health and healing.

5 Yoga Poses for Irritable Bowel Syndrome

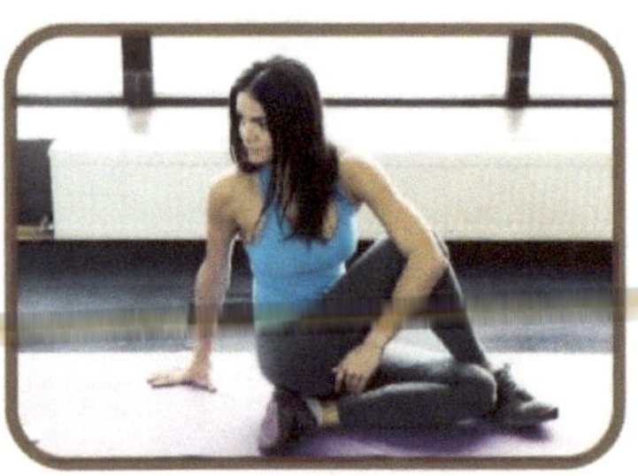

Ardha Matsyendrasana
(Lord of the Fishes Pose)

This pose has been found effective in relieving the symptoms of indigestion and constipation. It is also known to help improve metabolism, improve blood pressure and enhance the ability to adapt to stress.

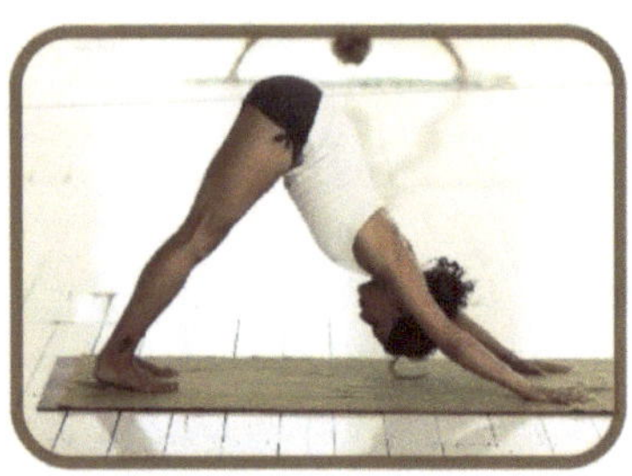

Adho Mukha Shvanasana
(Downward-facing Dog Pose)

This pose works in toning the abdominal muscles. It is also helpful in improving digestion and in boosting blood flow to the brain. This further helps in calming the mind and in energizing the body.

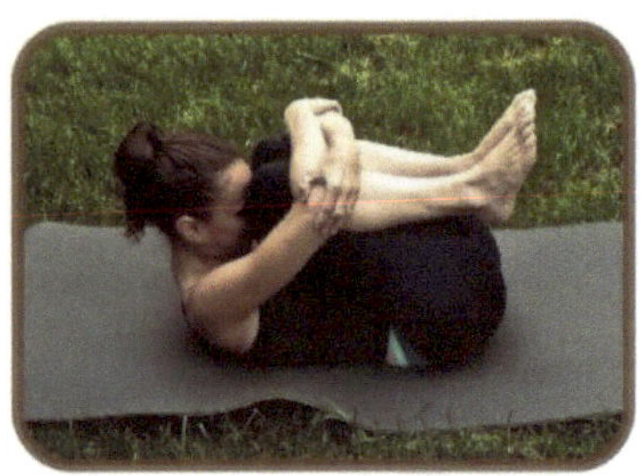

Pawanmuktasana
(Wind-relieving Pose)

This pose better enables the abdominal organs and intestines to be massaged. It is also helpful in releasing excess gas from the body while also improving digestion.

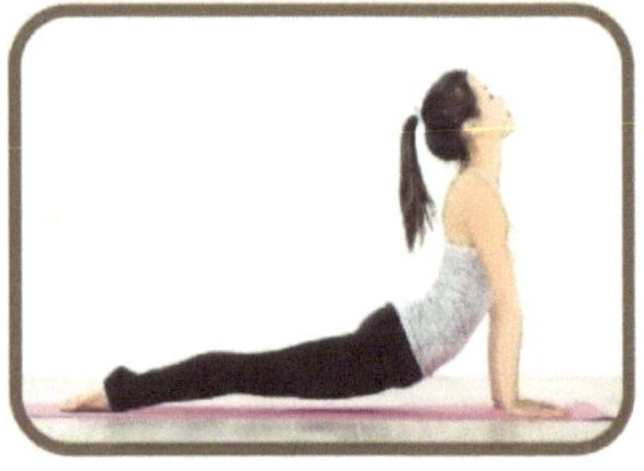

Bhujangasana
(Cobra Pose)

This is helpful in toning the abdomen, improving blood flow and lowering levels of stress. This pose also allows certain parts of the body to be stretched which is helpful in relieving fatigue and preventing strains.

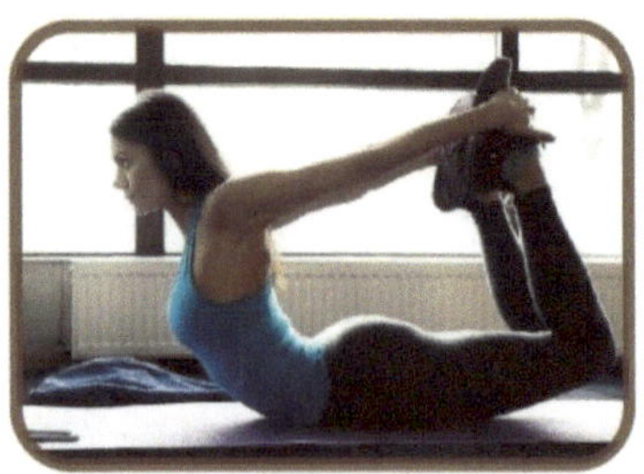

Dhanurasana Pose
(Bow Pose)

Dhanurasana is known to help relieve fatigue, stress, constipation and kidney disorders. It also improves intestinal function, appetite and digestion.

Use the FODMAPs Diet for Irritable Bowel Syndrome (IBS) Relief

If you suffer from IBS, have you heard of the low-FODMAP diet for relieving the associated symptoms?

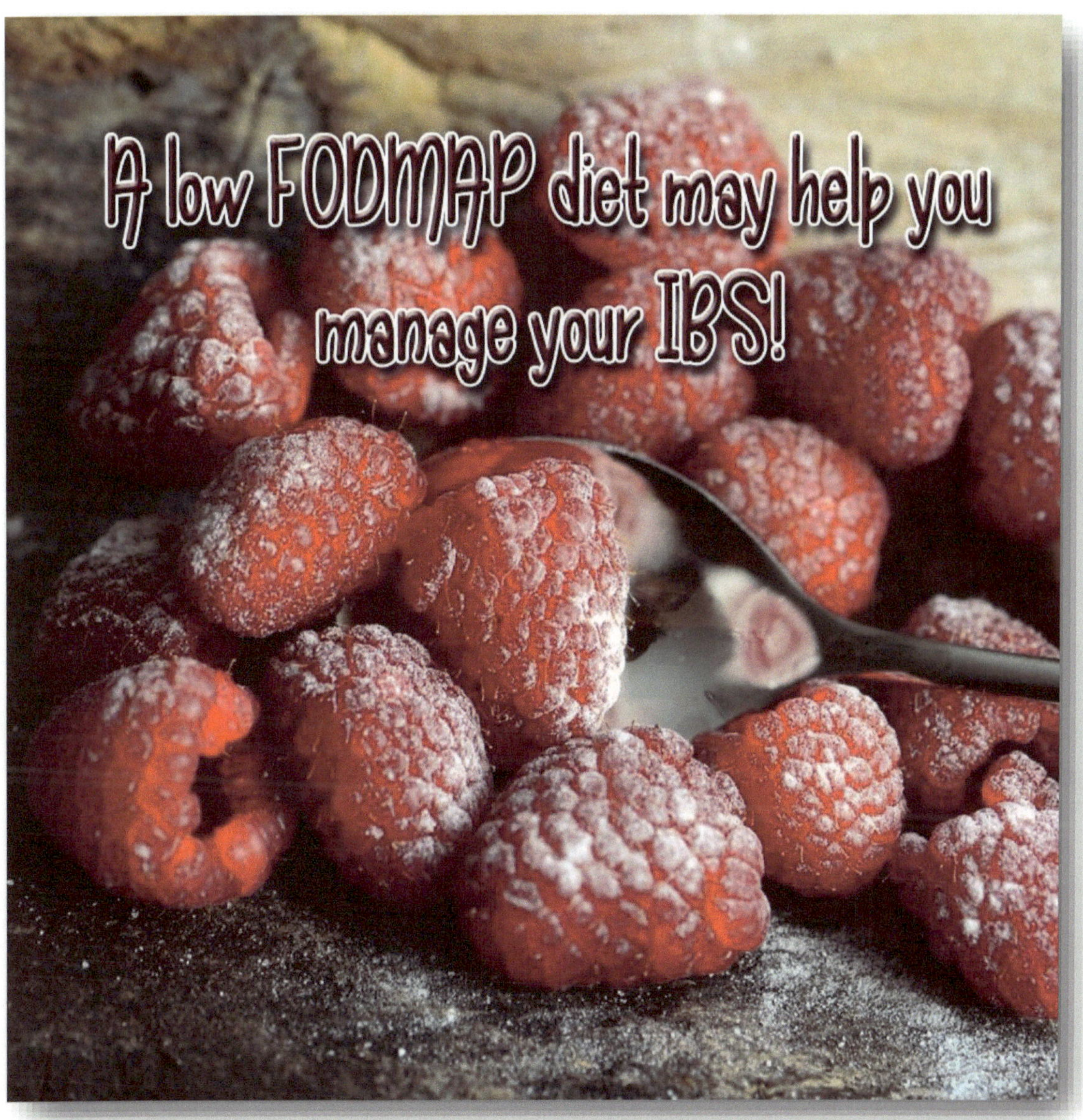

FODMAP is an acronym for:
- Fermentable Oligosaccharides
- Disaccharides
- Monosaccharides

- and Polyols

How Do FODMAPs Impact Irritable Bowel Syndrome

FODMAPs are sugars, found in the foods we eat, that may not be easy for some people to absorb. Poorly digested food that travels to the large intestine can ferment in the bowel and cause digestive stress.

Common FODMAPs found in some foods include most fruit and vegetables, nuts, cow's milk, legumes, artificial sweeteners and cereals. It is these foods, and similar others, that are believed to trigger symptoms of IBS.

It is now estimated that over 12% of the world population are sufferers of this condition. Of these, two thirds report that food is a contributing factor to their symptoms.

FODMAP Diet

A low FODMAP diet is not designed to be permanent. It is a temporary highly restrictive diet that lasts for several weeks. It identifies foods in the diet that trigger episodes of IBS. It restricts then slowly reintroduces FODMAP foods to the diet.

This diet restricts all FODMAP food from your diet at once, making it much more efficient than removing them one by one. When all FODMAPs are removed from the diet the gut can heal. Good bacteria are then able to correct any imbalances in the gut.

How the FODMAP Diet Works

For a period of three to eight weeks, you go through the elimination phase. The length of time depends on how you respond.

However, a minimum of three weeks is recommended so that your body has ample time, free of FODMAPs to adjust to more normalized gut flora ratios. During this phase all FODMAP food is eliminated from your diet.

Reintroduction Phase

After the elimination phase it is time to reintroduce FODMAP food back into your diet. This is done gradually by introducing food types one at a time. This allows you to see what food triggers unwanted symptoms. For example, add the fructose type of foods (a sugar found in fruit and some vegetables) to your diet, for one week.

If this results in you not having any IBS symptoms, you are ready to add another food type to your diet for one week. This could be lactose (a sugar found in dairy food). This process continues until you find out what food triggers your symptoms. This process allows you to eliminate the problem causing foods from your diet.

Because of food elimination, it is vital to ensure that important nutrients are not lacking in your diet. It is best to have assistance from and experienced dietitian to ensure your intake of vitamins is adequate. The ultimate goal of a low FODMAP diet is to achieve a balance.

High FODMAP foods that cause symptoms can be replaced by high FODMAP foods that you are able to tolerate. Individual FODMAP tolerance varies from person to person. Many find their diet does not have to be as strict as before. They can consume eliminated food occasionally but in smaller quantities.

Confirmed Results

In regulated studies involving irritable bowel syndrome patients and control groups of similar people without IBS, FODMAP restricted diets have proven to reduce overall IBS symptoms by 50%.

Up to 75% of study participants across many studies recorded an improvement in their symptoms. Noticeable improvements are observed one week after implementing the diet. Improvements were seen for bloating, abdominal pain, wind, and stool consistency.

Conclusion

Because the symptoms of IBS are centered on the digestive system, it is natural to lay the blame solely on physical causes, especially diet.

While this is certainly a probable factor, it is necessary to at least consider the mental and emotional inputs that may also be contributing to the problem and may even be the primary cause.

As with most conditions that have a lifestyle aspect, managing the underlying cause(s) will provide a better overall outcome than only focusing on the symptoms.

The symptoms of IBS are your body's feedback mechanism at work. Here it is telling you that *something is not quite right*.

Take the time to listen to what your body is trying to tell you. Usually, there is too much of something, rather than too little. Is it a food type, too much stress or anxiety, or a combination?

Take steady, positive action to remove the likely triggering influences and free yourself from the stressing symptoms of IBS.

About the Author

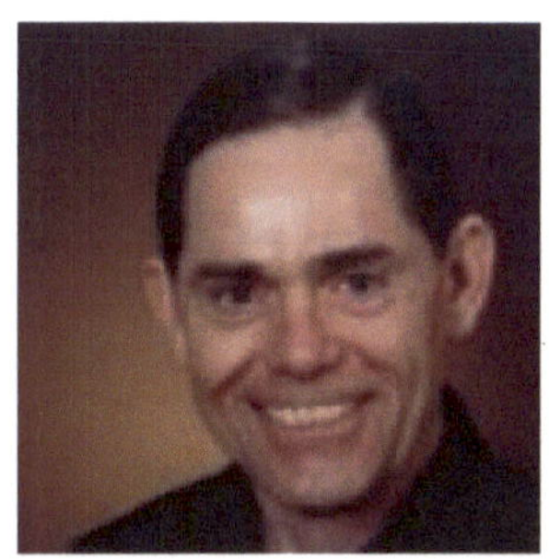

I have published numerous books on Amazon (both for Kindle and in paperback), along with other publishing platforms.

While most of my books are on health and fitness in general, I also write on baby boomer and older citizen health issues and have a recent interest in creating and printing journals/planners and other printable products.

Besides my own writing, I also ghostwrite ebooks, books, reports, articles, blogs and do Kindle conversions for clients on a variety of topics.

Today my wife and I are retired from our careers and live in Gold Canyon, AZ. I now write as a retirement business where you'll find me happily sitting in my office typing away on my laptop as I work on my next book or ghostwriting project . . . that is if we are not traveling on a cruise ship - our new-found mode of travel.